Vegan Fatty Liver Diet Cookbook

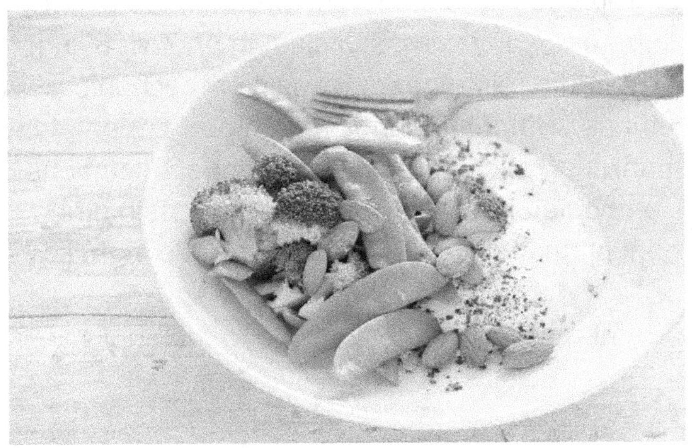

Nourishing Recipes for Healing and Health

Isaac Hendricks

Table of Contents

INTRODUCTION

In the realm of health and wellness, the significance of diet in managing various conditions cannot be overstated. Among the myriad health concerns, fatty liver disease stands as a prevalent and concerning issue, affecting millions worldwide. Fatty liver disease encompasses a spectrum of conditions ranging from simple steatosis to more severe forms like non-alcoholic steatohepatitis (NASH), often associated with obesity, insulin resistance, and metabolic syndrome.

This book is written for people who have fatty liver and are seeking a way to prevent it from getting worse, as well as individuals who are at risk of developing the disease. It is a resource that will help those with fatty liver disease plan their meals on a daily basis. It is not easy to find suitable meal plans and recipes because traditional diets for people with liver disease are not suitable for fatty liver. Trying to convert a fatty liver diet from a liver disease diet can be confusing, and most of the time the information is not tailored towards different stages of the disease.

This book also contains recipes that will be suitable for the varying degrees of fatty liver, the incidences of fatty liver disease that still can occur even in people with no symptoms of any liver abnormalities. These could be any person of any age. The beginning stages of fatty liver disease will be people looking to control and prevent their disease from getting worse. An increase in the levels of fatty liver disease has also been diagnosed for children. With the epidemic of childhood obesity, type II diabetes, and metabolic syndrome, there are quite a significant number of children and teenagers suffering from fatty liver. Steps to correct fatty liver and prevent the likelihood of severe consequences must be taken from an early age. This is also a resource for concerned parents and aspiring young individuals looking to turn around their health before it is too late.

While conventional wisdom often prescribes medication and lifestyle modifications such as weight loss and exercise to combat fatty liver disease, the role of diet, particularly a plant-based approach, is increasingly recognized as pivotal in ameliorating its effects. Enter the "Vegan Fatty Liver Diet Cookbook" – a comprehensive compendium of culinary solutions tailored to address the unique dietary needs of individuals grappling with fatty liver disease within the framework of a vegan lifestyle.

This cookbook represents more than just a collection of recipes; it symbolises a holistic approach to health, recognizing the intricate interplay between food, wellness, and disease management. Through the artful combination of wholesome, plant-based ingredients, carefully curated recipes, and evidence-based nutritional guidance, this cookbook endeavours to empower individuals on their journey toward liver health and overall well-being.

Within these pages, you will discover an array of delectable dishes thoughtfully crafted to support liver function, promote detoxification, reduce inflammation, and foster metabolic equilibrium – all while tantalising your taste buds and invigorating your culinary repertoire. From vibrant salads bursting with antioxidants to hearty mains brimming with plant-powered protein and fibre, each recipe is meticulously designed to not only nourish the body but also inspire a newfound appreciation for the rich tapestry of flavours inherent in plant-based cuisine.

Whether you are navigating the complexities of fatty liver disease for the first time or seeking innovative ways to optimise your dietary habits, this cookbook serves as your steadfast companion and trusted guide. Join us as we embark on a journey of culinary exploration and wellness enhancement, where every dish represents a step toward reclaiming vitality, vitality, and vitality. Together, let us harness the transformative power of food to cultivate a healthier, happier, and more vibrant existence.

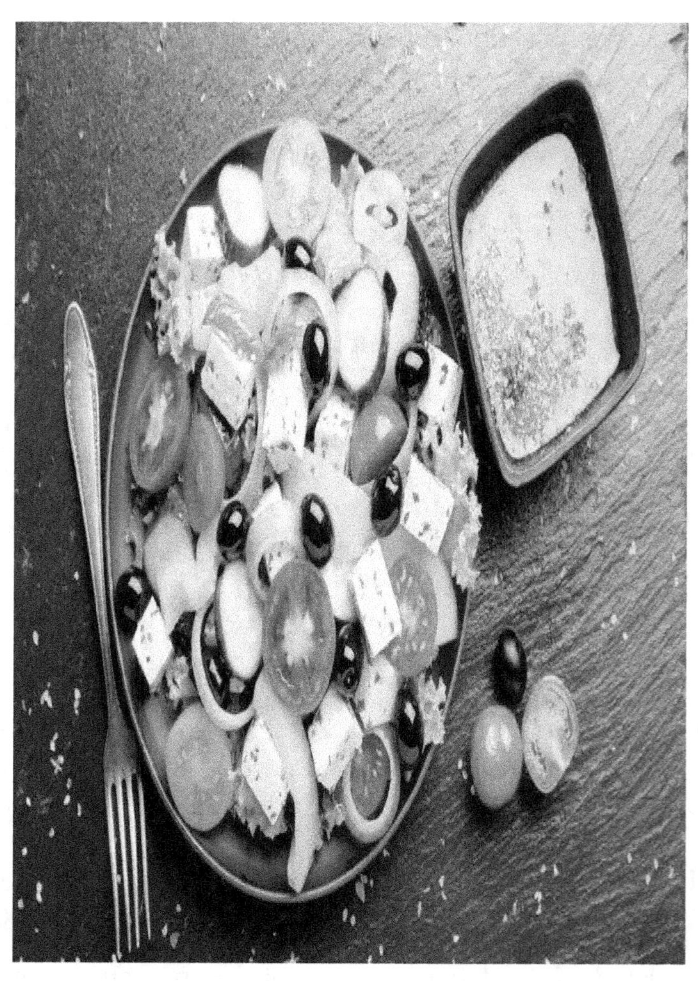

CHAPTER ONE

Understanding Fatty Liver Disease

What is Fatty Liver Disease?

Fatty liver disease, also known as hepatic steatosis, is a condition characterised by the accumulation of fat in the liver cells. While a small amount of fat in the liver is normal, excessive fat accumulation can lead to inflammation and liver damage.

Fatty liver disease is broadly categorised into two main types:
alcoholic and non-alcoholic (NAFLD).

1. Alcoholic Fatty Liver Disease (AFLD): As the name suggests, AFLD is caused by excessive alcohol consumption. The liver metabolises alcohol, and chronic alcohol abuse can lead to fat accumulation in liver cells, impairing liver function. AFLD can progress to more severe conditions such as alcoholic hepatitis and cirrhosis if alcohol consumption continues unabated.

2. Non-Alcoholic Fatty Liver Disease (NAFLD): NAFLD is the most common form of fatty liver disease and occurs in individuals who

do not consume excessive amounts of alcohol. It is often associated with obesity, insulin resistance, type 2 diabetes, high cholesterol, and metabolic syndrome. NAFLD ranges from simple fatty liver, which typically does not cause serious liver damage, to non-alcoholic steatohepatitis (NASH), a more severe form characterised by inflammation and liver cell damage. NASH can progress to advanced fibrosis, cirrhosis, and even liver cancer.

Risk factors for developing fatty liver disease include:

- Obesity: Excess body weight, particularly visceral fat around the abdomen, increases the risk of fat accumulation in the liver.

- Insulin Resistance and Type 2 Diabetes: Insulin resistance, a condition in which cells become resistant to the effects of insulin, and type 2 diabetes are closely linked to NAFLD.

- High Blood Pressure: Hypertension is associated with an increased risk of fatty liver disease.

- High Cholesterol and Triglycerides: Elevated levels of cholesterol and

triglycerides in the blood can contribute to
fat accumulation in the liver.

- Metabolic Syndrome: A cluster of conditions
  including obesity, high blood pressure, high
  blood sugar, and abnormal lipid levels,
  which collectively increase the risk of fatty
  liver disease.

- Rapid Weight Loss: Losing weight too
  quickly, especially through crash diets or
  bariatric surgery, can exacerbate liver fat
  accumulation.

Fatty liver disease often progresses silently, with
few or no symptoms in the early stages. However,
as the condition advances, individuals may
experience fatigue, abdominal discomfort,
weakness, jaundice (yellowing of the skin and
eyes), and complications such as liver fibrosis,
cirrhosis, and liver failure.

Early detection and lifestyle modifications, including
dietary changes, weight loss, regular exercise, and
avoidance of alcohol, are crucial in managing and
potentially reversing fatty liver disease. Seeking
medical advice and monitoring liver health through
regular screenings are essential steps in mitigating
the risks associated with this increasingly prevalent
condition.

Causes and Risk Factors

Fatty liver disease, whether alcoholic or non-alcoholic, results from a complex interplay of genetic, environmental, and lifestyle factors. Understanding the causes and risk factors associated with this condition is paramount in its prevention and management. While some factors, such as genetics, are beyond our control, many are modifiable through lifestyle interventions. Here, we delve into the causes and risk factors of fatty liver disease:

1. **Obesity:** Excess body weight, particularly visceral adipose tissue (fat around the abdomen), significantly increases the risk of developing fatty liver disease. Obesity is closely linked to insulin resistance, which promotes fat accumulation in the liver.

2. **Insulin Resistance and Type 2 Diabetes:** Insulin resistance, a condition in which cells fail to respond effectively to insulin, is a hallmark of type 2 diabetes and metabolic syndrome. Insulin resistance contributes to the accumulation of fat in the liver, a key feature of non-alcoholic fatty liver disease (NAFLD).

3. **High Blood Pressure (Hypertension):** Hypertension is associated with an increased risk of fatty liver disease,

particularly in individuals with metabolic syndrome. Elevated blood pressure can exacerbate liver damage and inflammation.

4. **High Cholesterol and Triglycerides:** Elevated levels of cholesterol and triglycerides in the blood are risk factors for fatty liver disease. Dyslipidemia, characterised by abnormal lipid levels, contributes to liver fat accumulation and inflammation.

5. **Metabolic Syndrome:** Metabolic syndrome is a cluster of conditions including obesity, insulin resistance, hypertension, and dyslipidemia, all of which increase the risk of developing fatty liver disease. The combination of these metabolic abnormalities significantly heightens the likelihood of liver fat accumulation and inflammation.

6. **Alcohol Consumption:** Excessive alcohol consumption is a primary cause of alcoholic fatty liver disease (AFLD). Chronic alcohol abuse can lead to fat accumulation in the liver, inflammation, and liver damage. The risk of AFLD increases with the quantity and duration of alcohol consumption.

7. **Rapid Weight Loss:** Losing weight too quickly, especially through crash diets or bariatric surgery, can exacerbate liver fat accumulation and increase the risk of developing fatty liver disease. Rapid weight loss leads to the release of fatty acids from adipose tissue, overwhelming the liver's capacity to metabolise them effectively.

8. **Genetics:** Genetic factors may predispose certain individuals to fatty liver disease. Variations in genes involved in lipid metabolism, insulin signalling, and inflammation can influence an individual's susceptibility to liver fat accumulation and disease progression.

9. **Sedentary Lifestyle:** Lack of physical activity is associated with an increased risk of developing fatty liver disease. Regular exercise helps improve insulin sensitivity, promote weight loss, and reduce liver fat accumulation.

10. **Dietary Factors:** Consumption of a diet high in refined carbohydrates, sugars, and saturated fats, along with low intake of fruits, vegetables, and fibre, is linked to an increased risk of fatty liver disease. Poor dietary habits contribute to obesity, insulin

resistance, and dyslipidemia, all of which promote liver fat accumulation.

Understanding these causes and risk factors empowers individuals to make informed lifestyle choices and adopt preventive measures to reduce their risk of fatty liver disease. By addressing modifiable risk factors through dietary modifications, weight management, regular exercise, and avoidance of excessive alcohol consumption, individuals can take proactive steps toward liver health and overall well-being.

Symptoms and Diagnosis

Fatty liver disease often progresses silently, with few or no noticeable symptoms in the early stages. As the condition advances, symptoms may become apparent, indicating liver damage and inflammation. Additionally, diagnosis typically involves a combination of medical history, physical examination, laboratory tests, imaging studies, and, in some cases, liver biopsy. Here's a closer look at the symptoms and diagnostic methods associated with fatty liver disease:

<u>**Symptoms:**</u>

1. **Fatigue:** Persistent fatigue and weakness are common symptoms of fatty liver disease, often attributed to impaired liver function and inflammation.

2. **Abdominal Discomfort:** Some individuals with fatty liver disease may experience discomfort or pain in the upper right abdomen, where the liver is located. This discomfort may be dull, achy, or intermittent.

3. **Weight Loss:** Unintentional weight loss may occur in individuals with advanced fatty liver disease, particularly in cases of non-alcoholic steatohepatitis (NASH) or cirrhosis.

4. **Jaundice:** In rare cases, jaundice may occur as a result of liver damage in advanced stages of fatty liver disease. Jaundice is characterised by yellowing of the skin and eyes, dark urine, and pale stools.

5. **Swelling:** Swelling of the abdomen (ascites) or lower extremities (edema) may occur in advanced stages of liver disease, indicating fluid retention.

6. **Mental Confusion:** In severe cases of liver disease, cognitive impairment or confusion (hepatic encephalopathy) may occur due to the liver's inability to detoxify harmful substances from the blood.

7. **Easy Bruising and Bleeding:** Impaired liver function can affect blood clotting, leading to easy bruising and bleeding tendencies.

Diagnosis:

1. **Medical History and Physical Examination:** A comprehensive medical history, including information about alcohol consumption, medications, and risk factors for fatty liver disease, is obtained. A physical examination may reveal signs such as an enlarged liver (hepatomegaly) or abdominal tenderness.

2. **Blood Tests:** Blood tests are used to assess liver function and screen for markers of liver damage and inflammation. Commonly ordered blood tests include liver enzyme tests (ALT, AST), markers of liver function (bilirubin, albumin), and tests for metabolic abnormalities (glucose, cholesterol, triglycerides).

3. **Imaging Studies:** Imaging techniques such as ultrasound, computed tomography (CT), or magnetic resonance imaging (MRI) may be used to visualise the liver and assess for signs of fat accumulation, inflammation, or liver damage. These imaging modalities can

help confirm the diagnosis of fatty liver disease and evaluate its severity.

4. **FibroScan:** FibroScan is a non-invasive imaging technique that measures liver stiffness, providing information about the degree of liver fibrosis (scarring) associated with fatty liver disease.

5. **Liver Biopsy:** In some cases, a liver biopsy may be performed to obtain a tissue sample for microscopic examination. A liver biopsy can provide valuable information about the extent of liver damage, inflammation, and fibrosis, guiding treatment decisions and prognosis.

Early detection and diagnosis of fatty liver disease are crucial for implementing appropriate management strategies and preventing disease progression. Individuals experiencing symptoms suggestive of liver dysfunction should seek prompt medical evaluation and undergo comprehensive diagnostic testing to assess liver health and determine the underlying cause of their symptoms.

Importance of Diet in Managing Fatty Liver

Diet plays a pivotal role in the management of fatty liver disease, offering a powerful tool for improving liver health, reducing inflammation, and potentially reversing liver damage. Adopting a well-balanced, nutrient-dense diet can help individuals with fatty liver disease mitigate risk factors, promote weight loss, improve insulin sensitivity, and optimise overall metabolic function. Here's a closer look at the importance of diet in managing fatty liver:

1. **Promotes Weight Loss:** Obesity and excess body weight are significant risk factors for fatty liver disease. A calorie-controlled diet rich in whole foods, fruits, vegetables, lean proteins, and healthy fats can support weight loss efforts, reduce visceral adiposity, and decrease fat accumulation in the liver.

2. **Reduces Liver Fat Accumulation:** Certain dietary patterns, such as the Mediterranean diet or a plant-based diet, have been shown to reduce liver fat accumulation and improve liver function in individuals with fatty liver disease. These diets emphasise whole grains, legumes, nuts, seeds, fruits, vegetables, and healthy fats while limiting processed foods, added sugars, and saturated fats.

3. **Improves Insulin Sensitivity:** Insulin resistance is a key driver of fatty liver disease, particularly in cases of non-alcoholic fatty liver disease (NAFLD). Dietary strategies that promote stable blood

sugar levels, such as consuming complex carbohydrates, fibre-rich foods, and lean proteins, can improve insulin sensitivity and reduce the risk of NAFLD progression.

4. **Lowers Inflammation:** Chronic inflammation plays a central role in the pathogenesis of fatty liver disease and its progression to more severe forms such as non-alcoholic steatohepatitis (NASH) and liver fibrosis. Anti-inflammatory diets rich in antioxidants, omega-3 fatty acids, and phytonutrients can help mitigate inflammation and protect against liver damage.

5. **Supports Liver Detoxification:** The liver plays a crucial role in detoxifying harmful substances from the body. Certain foods and nutrients, such as cruciferous vegetables (e.g., broccoli, kale, Brussels sprouts), sulphur-containing compounds, and antioxidants (e.g., vitamin C, glutathione), support liver detoxification pathways, enhancing the liver's ability to eliminate toxins and metabolic waste products.

6. **Optimises Nutrient Intake:** Nutrient deficiencies, including vitamins (e.g., vitamin D, vitamin E) and minerals (e.g., magnesium, zinc), are common in

individuals with fatty liver disease and may contribute to disease progression. A well-balanced diet that provides adequate micronutrients supports liver health, immune function, and overall well-being.

7. **Prevents Complications:** Managing fatty liver disease through dietary interventions can help prevent complications such as liver fibrosis, cirrhosis, and liver cancer. By addressing underlying risk factors and promoting liver health, dietary modifications reduce the likelihood of disease progression and improve long-term outcomes.

8. **Enhances Quality of Life:** Adopting a healthy diet not only benefits liver health but also contributes to overall vitality, energy levels, and quality of life. By nourishing the body with wholesome, nutrient-rich foods, individuals with fatty liver disease can experience improved physical health, mental well-being, and resilience.

In conclusion, diet plays a central role in the management of fatty liver disease, offering a safe, effective, and sustainable approach to improving liver health and overall well-being. By embracing dietary modifications that prioritise whole foods, promote weight loss, reduce inflammation, and support liver function, individuals can take proactive steps toward managing their condition and optimising their health for the long term.

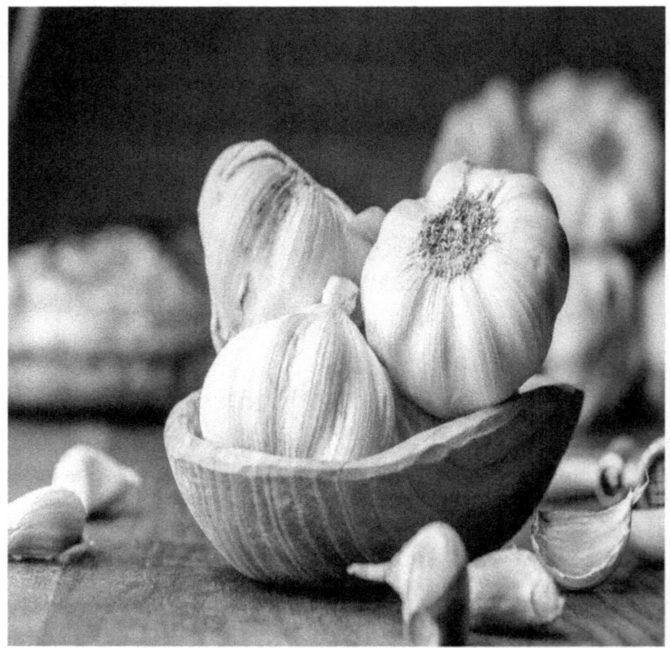

CHAPTER TWO

The Basics of Vegan Nutrition

Key Nutrients for a Healthy Vegan Diet

Following a vegan diet can offer numerous health benefits, including reduced risk of chronic diseases such as heart disease, diabetes, and certain cancers. However, it's essential to ensure that a vegan diet is well-balanced and provides all the necessary nutrients for optimal health, especially when managing conditions like fatty liver disease. Here are some key nutrients to focus on when following a vegan diet for liver health:

1. **Omega-3 Fatty Acids:** Omega-3 fatty acids, particularly EPA (eicosapentaenoic acid) and DHA (docosahexaenoic acid), play a crucial role in reducing inflammation and supporting liver health. While these fatty acids are commonly found in fatty fish, vegans can obtain them from plant-based sources such as flaxseeds, chia seeds, hemp seeds, walnuts, and algae-based supplements.

2. **Antioxidants:** Antioxidants help protect the liver from oxidative stress and inflammation, which are key contributors to fatty liver disease. Colourful fruits and vegetables are

rich in antioxidants such as vitamin C, vitamin E, beta-carotene, and flavonoids. Include a variety of berries, citrus fruits, leafy greens, bell peppers, tomatoes, and cruciferous vegetables in your diet to maximise antioxidant intake.

3. **Fibre:** Dietary fibre plays a crucial role in promoting digestive health, regulating blood sugar levels, and supporting weight management. Fibre-rich foods such as whole grains, legumes, fruits, vegetables, nuts, and seeds help maintain satiety, stabilise blood sugar levels, and promote healthy gut microbiota, which is essential for liver health.

4. **Plant-Based Proteins:** Protein is essential for supporting liver function, repairing tissues, and maintaining muscle mass. While animal products are a common source of protein, vegans can meet their protein needs by incorporating plant-based sources such as beans, lentils, chickpeas, tofu, tempeh, seitan, quinoa, nuts, and seeds into their diet.

5. **B Vitamins:** B vitamins, including folate (B9), B6, and B12, play vital roles in energy metabolism, DNA synthesis, and liver function. While plant-based foods naturally contain folate and B6, vitamin B12 is

primarily found in fortified foods or supplements for vegans. Include fortified plant milks, breakfast cereals, nutritional yeast, and B12 supplements to ensure adequate intake.

6. **Iron:** Iron is essential for the production of red blood cells and oxygen transport throughout the body. Plant-based sources of iron include legumes, tofu, tempeh, soybeans, lentils, fortified cereals, quinoa, pumpkin seeds, and dark leafy greens. Consuming vitamin C-rich foods alongside iron-rich foods enhances iron absorption.

7. **Calcium:** Calcium is crucial for bone health, muscle function, and nerve transmission. While dairy products are traditional sources of calcium, vegans can obtain calcium from fortified plant milks, fortified orange juice, tofu made with calcium sulphate, almonds, sesame seeds, tahini, kale, collard greens, and broccoli.

8. **Vitamin D:** Vitamin D plays a role in immune function, bone health, and mood regulation. While sunlight exposure is a primary source of vitamin D, vegans may need to rely on fortified foods (e.g., plant-based milks, breakfast cereals, orange juice) or vitamin D supplements, particularly if sunlight exposure is limited.

By prioritising these key nutrients in a well-planned vegan diet, individuals can support liver health, reduce inflammation, and optimise overall well-being. Incorporating a diverse array of nutrient-rich plant foods and, if necessary, fortified foods or supplements ensures that vegans can meet their nutritional needs for optimal liver function and disease management.

Tips for Meeting Nutritional Needs on a Vegan Diet

1. **Eat a Variety of Foods:** Consuming a diverse array of plant-based foods ensures that you obtain a wide range of nutrients. Include fruits, vegetables, whole grains, legumes, nuts, seeds, and plant-based protein sources in your diet to maximise nutrient intake.

2. **Focus on Whole Foods:** Whole, minimally processed foods are rich in essential nutrients and fibre. Prioritise whole grains (e.g., brown rice, quinoa, oats), fresh fruits and vegetables, legumes, nuts, and seeds over highly processed vegan alternatives.

3. **Plan Balanced Meals:** Aim to include a source of protein, carbohydrates, healthy fats, and plenty of vegetables in each meal. For example, pair beans or tofu with whole

grains and leafy greens for a balanced meal
that provides protein, fibre, vitamins, and
minerals.

4. **Include Protein-Rich Foods:** Incorporate a
    variety of plant-based protein sources such
    as beans, lentils, chickpeas, tofu, tempeh,
    seitan, quinoa, nuts, and seeds into your
    meals and snacks to meet your protein
    needs.

5. **Don't Forget Omega-3s:** Include
    plant-based sources of omega-3 fatty acids,
    such as flaxseeds, chia seeds, hemp seeds,
    walnuts, and algae-based supplements, to
    support heart and brain health.

6. **Consume Calcium-Rich Foods:** Ensure
    adequate calcium intake by including
    calcium-fortified plant milks, fortified orange
    juice, tofu made with calcium sulphate,
    almonds, sesame seeds, tahini, and dark
    leafy greens (e.g., kale, collard greens, bok
    choy) in your diet.

7. **Opt for Iron-Rich Foods:** Incorporate
    iron-rich plant foods such as legumes, tofu,
    tempeh, soybeans, lentils, fortified cereals,
    quinoa, pumpkin seeds, and dark leafy
    greens to support healthy red blood cell
    production.

8. **Pair Iron-Rich Foods with Vitamin C:** Enhance iron absorption by consuming vitamin C-rich foods alongside iron-rich foods. For example, add citrus fruits, bell peppers, tomatoes, or broccoli to iron-containing meals.

9. **Consider Vitamin B12 Supplementation:** Since vitamin B12 is primarily found in animal products, vegans may need to supplement with B12-fortified foods or supplements to prevent deficiency. Choose fortified plant milks, breakfast cereals, nutritional yeast, or B12 supplements to meet your needs.

10. **Get Adequate Sun Exposure or Supplement Vitamin D:** If sunlight exposure is limited, consider taking a vitamin D supplement to maintain adequate levels. Alternatively, consume fortified foods such as plant-based milks, breakfast cereals, or orange juice to boost vitamin D intake.

11. **Read Labels:** When purchasing packaged foods, check labels for hidden animal-derived ingredients and additives. Look for vegan-certified or plant-based alternatives whenever possible.

12. **Consult a Registered Dietitian:** If you're
   unsure about meeting your nutritional needs
   on a vegan diet, consider consulting a
   registered dietitian with expertise in
   plant-based nutrition. They can provide
   personalised guidance and meal planning
   tips to ensure you meet your nutrient
   requirements.

By following these tips and adopting a well-planned
vegan diet that emphasises whole, nutrient-rich
foods, you can easily meet your nutritional needs
while enjoying the benefits of a plant-based
lifestyle.

Common Nutrient Deficiencies and How to Avoid Them

While a well-planned vegan diet can provide ample
nutrients, certain micronutrients may be more
challenging to obtain solely from plant-based
sources. Being aware of common nutrient
deficiencies and taking proactive steps to address
them can help ensure optimal health on a vegan
diet.
Here are some common nutrient deficiencies and
strategies to avoid them:

1. **Vitamin B12:** Vitamin B12 is primarily found
   in animal products, making it a critical

nutrient for vegans to pay attention to. Deficiency in vitamin B12 can lead to fatigue, weakness, nerve damage, and anaemia. To avoid deficiency, incorporate fortified foods such as plant-based milks, breakfast cereals, nutritional yeast, or take a B12 supplement regularly.

2. **Calcium:** While calcium is abundant in dairy products, vegans need to seek out alternative sources to maintain bone health. Include calcium-fortified plant milks, fortified orange juice, tofu made with calcium sulphate, almonds, sesame seeds, tahini, and dark leafy greens (e.g., kale, collard greens, bok choy) in your diet to meet calcium needs.

3. **Vitamin D:** Vitamin D is essential for bone health, immune function, and mood regulation. Since few foods naturally contain vitamin D, and sunlight exposure may be limited, consider taking a vitamin D supplement or consuming fortified foods such as plant-based milks, breakfast cereals, or orange juice to ensure adequate intake.

4. **Omega-3 Fatty Acids:** Omega-3 fatty acids, particularly EPA and DHA, are important for heart and brain health. While fatty fish is a common source of these fatty

acids, vegans can obtain them from plant-based sources such as flaxseeds, chia seeds, hemp seeds, walnuts, and algae-based supplements.

5. **Iron:** Iron is essential for the production of red blood cells and oxygen transport throughout the body. Plant-based sources of iron include legumes, tofu, tempeh, soybeans, lentils, fortified cereals, quinoa, pumpkin seeds, and dark leafy greens. Enhance iron absorption by consuming vitamin C-rich foods alongside iron-rich foods.

6. **Zinc:** Zinc plays a crucial role in immune function, wound healing, and DNA synthesis. Plant-based sources of zinc include legumes, tofu, tempeh, nuts, seeds, whole grains, and fortified cereals. Soaking, sprouting, or fermenting grains and legumes can improve zinc absorption.

7. **Iodine:** Iodine is essential for thyroid health and cognitive function. Sea vegetables such as nori, kombu, and wakame are excellent sources of iodine. If sea vegetables are not regularly consumed, consider using iodized salt or taking an iodine supplement to ensure adequate intake.

8. **Protein:** While protein deficiency is rare on a well-planned vegan diet, it's essential to consume a variety of protein-rich plant foods to meet protein needs. Include beans, lentils, chickpeas, tofu, tempeh, seitan, quinoa, nuts, and seeds in your diet to ensure adequate protein intake.

By incorporating a diverse array of nutrient-rich plant foods, including fortified foods and supplements when necessary, vegans can easily meet their nutritional needs and enjoy the health benefits of a plant-based lifestyle. Regularly monitoring nutrient intake and consulting with a registered dietitian can provide personalised guidance to address individual nutrient concerns and optimise overall health on a vegan diet.

CHAPTER THREE

Vegan Diet and Fatty Liver Disease

The Link Between Veganism and Liver Health
Veganism is a lifestyle that abstains from the consumption of animal products, including meat, dairy, eggs, and other animal-derived ingredients. Instead, it focuses on plant-based foods such as fruits, vegetables, grains, legumes, nuts, and seeds. The core principles of veganism extend beyond dietary choices to encompass ethical, environmental, and health considerations.

Understanding Liver Health: The Importance of a Healthy Liver
The liver is a vital organ responsible for numerous essential functions in the body, including metabolising nutrients, detoxifying harmful substances, producing bile for digestion, and storing glycogen for energy. Maintaining optimal liver health is crucial for overall well-being, as it directly impacts digestion, metabolism, immune function, and detoxification processes.
The Impact of Diet on Liver Health: How Food Choices Matter
Diet plays a significant role in liver health, as the liver processes the nutrients and substances absorbed from the foods we consume. Certain

dietary habits, such as excessive consumption of saturated fats, refined sugars, and processed foods, can contribute to liver damage and increase the risk of developing liver conditions such as fatty liver disease, inflammation, and cirrhosis.

The Vegan Advantage: Plant-Powered Nutrition for Liver Wellness
A well-planned vegan diet can offer several benefits for liver health. Plant-based foods are rich in essential nutrients, antioxidants, fibre, and phytonutrients that support liver function and promote overall health. Studies have shown that vegan diets are associated with lower levels of liver fat, reduced inflammation, improved insulin sensitivity, and a decreased risk of developing fatty liver disease compared to omnivorous diets.

Research Insights: Studies on Veganism and Liver Health
Scientific research has provided valuable insights into the relationship between veganism and liver health. Studies have demonstrated that adopting a vegan diet can lead to improvements in liver enzymes, lipid profiles, and markers of liver inflammation and fibrosis. Additionally, plant-based diets have been shown to lower the risk of non-alcoholic fatty liver disease (NAFLD) and other liver-related conditions.

Practical Tips for Supporting Liver Health on a Vegan Diet

To support liver health on a vegan diet, it's essential to focus on consuming a diverse array of nutrient-dense plant foods. Incorporating foods rich in antioxidants, such as berries, leafy greens, cruciferous vegetables, and herbs like turmeric and ginger, can help protect the liver from oxidative stress and inflammation. Additionally, emphasising whole grains, legumes, nuts, seeds, and healthy fats like avocado and olive oil can provide essential nutrients and support liver function.
Conclusion: Harnessing the Power of Veganism for a Healthy Liver

In conclusion, the link between veganism and liver health is evident, with plant-based nutrition offering numerous benefits for supporting liver function and preventing liver-related conditions. By adopting a well-balanced vegan diet rich in whole plant foods, individuals can nourish their livers and promote overall health and vitality. Embracing the principles of veganism not only benefits individual health but also contributes to a more sustainable and compassionate world.

This comprehensive exploration highlights the potential of veganism as a dietary approach for promoting liver wellness and overall health.

Foods to Include in a Vegan Fatty Liver Diet

1. Fruits and Vegetables

- High in fibre, vitamins, minerals, and antioxidants.
- Include a variety of colourful fruits and vegetables such as berries, citrus fruits, leafy greens, cruciferous vegetables, and bell peppers.
- Aim for at least 5 servings per day to support liver health and overall well-being.

2. Whole Grains

- Excellent sources of complex carbohydrates, fibre, and B vitamins.
- Choose whole grains such as quinoa, brown rice, barley, oats, whole wheat, and bulgur.
- Incorporate whole grains into meals to provide sustained energy and support digestive health.

3. Legumes

- Rich in protein, fibre, vitamins, and minerals.
- Include beans, lentils, chickpeas, peas, and soy products like tofu and tempeh.

- Incorporate legumes into soups, salads, stews, and stir-fries for a nutritious and satisfying meal.

4. Healthy Fats

- Opt for sources of healthy fats that support liver health and reduce inflammation.
- Include foods rich in omega-3 fatty acids such as flaxseeds, chia seeds, hemp seeds, walnuts, and algae-based supplements.
- Use plant-based oils like olive oil, avocado oil, and coconut oil in moderation for cooking and dressing salads.

5. Nuts and Seeds

- Provide essential nutrients, healthy fats, protein, and antioxidants.
- Incorporate a variety of nuts and seeds such as almonds, cashews, pumpkin seeds, sunflower seeds, and sesame seeds into meals and snacks.
- Enjoy nut butters and seed spreads as a nutritious topping for toast, oatmeal, or fruit.

6. Herbs and Spices

- Enhance the flavour of dishes without adding excess salt or fat.

- Include herbs and spices with liver-supportive properties such as turmeric, ginger, garlic, cinnamon, cumin, and parsley.
- Experiment with different flavour combinations to make meals more enjoyable and satisfying.

7. Plant-Based Protein Sources

- Choose a variety of plant-based protein sources to meet daily protein needs.
- Incorporate protein-rich foods such as tofu, tempeh, seitan, edamame, quinoa, lentils, and black beans into meals.
- Combine complementary protein sources to ensure adequate protein intake and promote muscle health.

8. Herbal Teas and Infusions

- Hydrate with herbal teas and infusions that support liver health and aid digestion.
- Choose caffeine-free options such as dandelion root tea, green tea, peppermint tea, ginger tea, and chamomile tea.
- Enjoy herbal teas as a soothing beverage between meals or as part of a relaxing evening ritual.

By including these nutrient-rich foods in a vegan fatty liver diet, individuals can nourish their bodies, support liver function, and promote overall health and well-being. Remember to prioritise whole, minimally processed foods and maintain a balanced diet to optimise liver health and prevent liver-related conditions.

This guide provides a comprehensive list of foods suitable for a vegan fatty liver diet, focusing on nutrient-rich plant-based options to support liver health and overall well-being.

Foods to Avoid or Limit

Maintaining a healthy liver on a vegan diet involves not only choosing nutritious foods but also avoiding or limiting certain foods that can contribute to liver damage or inflammation. Here are some foods to be mindful of:

1. Processed Foods
   - Highly processed foods often contain additives, preservatives, and unhealthy fats that can burden the liver.
   - Limit intake of packaged snacks, fast food, sugary cereals, and convenience meals.

2. Added Sugars
   - Excessive sugar consumption can contribute to fatty liver disease and insulin resistance.

- Avoid sugary beverages like soda, fruit juices with added sugars, candy, and pastries.
- Opt for natural sweeteners like stevia, maple syrup, or dates in moderation.

3. Highly Refined Carbohydrates
- Foods made with white flour and refined grains lack fibre and essential nutrients.
- Minimise consumption of white bread, white rice, pasta, and baked goods made with refined flour.

4. Saturated and Trans Fats
- Saturated and trans fats can increase cholesterol levels and promote inflammation in the liver.
- Limit consumption of fried foods, fatty cuts of meat, butter, margarine, and hydrogenated oils.

5. Excessive Salt
- Consuming too much salt can lead to fluid retention and high blood pressure, putting strain on the liver.
- Avoid processed foods with high sodium content, such as canned soups, chips, and processed meats.
- Use herbs, spices, and lemon juice to flavour dishes instead of salt.

6. Alcohol
- Alcohol is a leading cause of liver damage and should be avoided entirely or consumed in moderation.
- Opt for alcohol-free beverages such as sparkling water with lemon or herbal teas.

7. Artificial Sweeteners and Additives
- Some artificial sweeteners and food additives may have negative effects on liver health.
- Limit consumption of artificial sweeteners like aspartame, saccharin, and sucralose, as well as artificial food colorings and flavourings.

8. Highly Processed Plant-Based Foods
- While plant-based alternatives can be convenient, some highly processed vegan foods may contain unhealthy additives and excess salt or sugar.
- Choose whole food plant-based options whenever possible and read labels carefully to avoid hidden additives.

By being mindful of these foods and making healthier choices, individuals can support liver health and enhance the effectiveness of a vegan fatty liver diet. Prioritising whole, nutrient-rich foods and minimising intake of processed and unhealthy options can contribute to overall well-being and vitality.

This section provides practical guidance on foods to avoid or limit for optimal liver health on a vegan diet, helping readers make informed choices to support their dietary goals and promote liver wellness.

CHAPTER FOUR

Meal Planning for Fatty Liver Health

Tips for Meal Planning on a Vegan Diet

1. **Balance Macronutrients:** Ensure each meal includes a balance of carbohydrates, protein, and healthy fats to provide sustained energy and promote overall health. Incorporate sources like legumes, tofu, tempeh, nuts, seeds, whole grains, and avocados.

2. **Include a Variety of Foods:** Aim for a diverse range of fruits, vegetables, grains, legumes, nuts, and seeds to obtain a wide array of essential nutrients. Incorporating different colours and textures also adds interest to meals.

3. **Plan Ahead:** Dedicate some time each week to plan your meals, including breakfast, lunch, dinner, and snacks. Consider factors like nutritional balance, convenience, and any dietary preferences or restrictions.

4. **Batch Cooking:** Prepare large batches of staples such as grains, beans, and roasted vegetables ahead of time. This makes it easier to throw together quick and nutritious meals throughout the week.

5. **Embrace Leftovers:** Cook larger portions and intentionally plan for leftovers. Leftover grains, proteins, and vegetables can be repurposed into new dishes or enjoyed as quick and easy lunches.

6. **Use a Meal Planning Template:** Utilise a meal planning template or app to organise your weekly meals. This can help you stay on track, avoid food waste, and ensure you're meeting your nutritional needs.

7. **Shop Wisely:** Make a grocery list based on your meal plan to avoid unnecessary purchases and reduce food waste. Focus on purchasing fresh, whole foods and minimise reliance on processed vegan products.

8. **Experiment with New Recipes:** Keep mealtime exciting by trying out new vegan recipes regularly. Look for inspiration from cookbooks, online resources, or vegan cooking blogs.

9. **Consider Nutrient Supplements:**
   Depending on your individual needs and
   dietary habits, you may benefit from
   supplementing certain nutrients commonly
   found in animal products, such as vitamin
   B12, vitamin D, and omega-3 fatty acids.

10. **Stay Flexible:** Be open to adjusting your
    meal plan based on changes in schedule,
    ingredient availability, or personal
    preferences. Flexibility is key to maintaining
    a sustainable and enjoyable vegan lifestyle.

Sample Meal Plans for Breakfast, Lunch, and Dinner

Here are sample meal plans for breakfast, lunch, and dinner for a vegan fatty liver diet:

Breakfast:
1. Quinoa Breakfast Bowl:

   - Ingredients:
     - Cooked quinoa
     - Sautéed spinach
     - Diced tomatoes
     - Sliced avocado
     - Toasted pumpkin seeds

- Instructions:
    - Combine cooked quinoa with sautéed spinach and diced tomatoes.
    - Top with sliced avocado and toasted pumpkin seeds for added texture and flavour.

2. Chia Seed Pudding:

- Ingredients:
    - Chia seeds
    - Almond milk
    - Mixed berries
    - Sliced almonds
    - Maple syrup (optional)

- Instructions:
    - Mix chia seeds with almond milk and let it sit in the refrigerator overnight to thicken.
    - Serve topped with mixed berries, sliced almonds, and a drizzle of maple syrup if desired.

Lunch:

1. Mediterranean Chickpea Salad:

- Ingredients:
    - Cooked chickpeas
    - Chopped cucumber
    - Diced bell peppers
    - Cherry tomatoes
    - Kalamata olives
    - Chopped parsley
    - Lemon-tahini dressing

- Instructions:
    - Combine chickpeas, cucumber, bell peppers, tomatoes, olives, and parsley in a bowl.
    - Drizzle with lemon-tahini dressing and toss to coat evenly.

2. Vegetable Stir-Fry with Tofu:

- Ingredients:
    - Cubed tofu
    - Mixed vegetables (such as bell peppers, broccoli, carrots, and snap peas)
    - Soy sauce
    - Garlic
    - Ginger
    - Brown rice or quinoa (optional)

- o Instructions:
    - ■ Sauté cubed tofu with garlic and ginger until golden brown.
    - ■ Add mixed vegetables and stir-fry until tender-crisp.
    - ■ Season with soy sauce and serve over brown rice or quinoa if desired.

Dinner:

1. Lentil and Sweet Potato Curry:

   - o Ingredients:
       - ■ Cooked lentils
       - ■ Diced sweet potatoes
       - ■ Chopped onion
       - ■ Minced garlic
       - ■ Curry powder
       - ■ Coconut milk
       - ■ Fresh cilantro

   - o Instructions:
       - ■ Sauté onion and garlic until softened.
       - ■ Add diced sweet potatoes and curry powder, then cook until fragrant.

- Stir in cooked lentils and coconut milk, then simmer until sweet potatoes are tender.
        - Serve garnished with fresh cilantro.

2. Stuffed Bell Peppers:

   - Ingredients:
     - Quinoa
     - Black beans
     - Corn kernels
     - Diced tomatoes
     - Chopped onion
     - Taco seasoning
     - Bell peppers

   - Instructions:
     - Cook quinoa according to package instructions.
     - In a skillet, sauté onion until translucent, then add black beans, corn, diced tomatoes, and taco seasoning.
     - Stir in cooked quinoa and mix well.
     - Stuff the mixture into halved bell peppers and bake until peppers are tender.

These sample meal plans offer a variety of nutrient-dense, plant-based options to support a vegan fatty liver diet. Adjust portions and ingredients as needed to suit individual preferences and nutritional requirements.

Healthy Snack Ideas

Here are some healthy snack ideas suitable for a vegan fatty liver diet:

1. **Raw Vegetable Sticks with Hummus:** Slice up crunchy vegetables like carrots, cucumbers, bell peppers, and celery and serve with a side of homemade or store-bought hummus. This snack is rich in fibre, vitamins, and minerals, and the hummus provides protein and healthy fats.

2. **Mixed Nuts and Seeds:** Create a custom mix of raw or roasted nuts and seeds such as almonds, walnuts, pumpkin seeds, and sunflower seeds. Nuts and seeds are excellent sources of healthy fats, protein, and essential nutrients like magnesium and zinc.

3. **Fresh Fruit with Nut Butter:** Pair slices of apple, banana, or pear with a dollop of almond butter, peanut butter, or cashew butter. This combination offers a balance of

natural sugars, fibre, and protein, making it a satisfying and nourishing snack.

4. **Edamame:** Enjoy a handful of steamed edamame pods sprinkled with a pinch of sea salt. Edamame is a great source of plant-based protein, fibre, and antioxidants, and it makes for a convenient and nutritious snack option.

5. **Chia Seed Pudding:** Whip up a batch of chia seed pudding by mixing chia seeds with almond milk and letting it thicken in the refrigerator. Serve topped with fresh berries or sliced fruit for added flavour and nutritional benefits.

6. **Roasted Chickpeas:** Season cooked chickpeas with your favourite herbs and spices, then roast them in the oven until crispy. Roasted chickpeas are a crunchy and satisfying snack packed with fibre, protein, and essential minerals like iron and manganese.

7. **Seaweed Snacks:** Enjoy the salty crunch of roasted seaweed sheets, which are low in calories and rich in vitamins and minerals, including iodine and iron. Look for varieties seasoned with natural ingredients like sesame oil and sea salt.

8. **Rice Cake with Avocado and Tomato:**
    Spread mashed avocado onto a rice cake
    and top with sliced tomato and a sprinkle of
    black pepper. Rice cakes provide a light and
    crispy base, while avocado adds creamy
    texture and healthy fats, and tomato offers
    freshness and flavour.

9. **Trail Mix:** Create your own trail mix by
    combining dried fruits like raisins or apricots
    with nuts, seeds, and a handful of dark
    chocolate chips or cacao nibs. This portable
    snack is perfect for satisfying cravings while
    providing a mix of carbohydrates, protein,
    and antioxidants.

10. **Vegetable Sushi Rolls:** Roll up nori sheets
    filled with thinly sliced vegetables like
    cucumber, avocado, and bell pepper, along
    with cooked brown rice or quinoa. Vegetable
    sushi rolls are a nutritious and satisfying
    snack option that's also fun to make at
    home.

CHAPTER FIVE

Delicious Vegan Breakfast Recipes

Green Smoothie Bowl

A Green Smoothie Bowl is a vibrant and nutrient-packed breakfast or snack option that's as delicious as it is healthy. Here's how to create your own:

Ingredients:

- 1 ripe banana, frozen
- 1 cup fresh spinach or kale
- 1/2 cup frozen pineapple chunks
- 1/2 cup frozen mango chunks
- 1/2 cup almond milk or any plant-based milk
- Toppings: sliced fruits (such as berries, kiwi, or banana), granola, nuts, seeds, coconut flakes, chia seeds, hemp hearts, etc.

Instructions:

1. Blend the Smoothie Base:
   - In a blender, combine the frozen banana, fresh spinach or kale, frozen pineapple chunks, frozen mango chunks, and almond milk.

- ○ Blend until smooth and creamy. You may need to stop and scrape down the sides of the blender to ensure all ingredients are well blended.

2. Pour into a Bowl:
   - ○ Once the smoothie base is well blended, pour it into a bowl. The consistency should be thick enough to hold the toppings.

3. Add Toppings:
   - ○ Arrange your desired toppings on top of the green smoothie base. Get creative with your choices to add flavour, texture, and extra nutrients.
   - ○ You can arrange toppings in sections or sprinkle them evenly across the bowl for a visually appealing presentation.

4. Enjoy:
   - ○ Grab a spoon and dive into your delicious creation! Mix the smoothie base with the toppings as you enjoy each spoonful.

Tips:

- Experiment with different combinations of fruits and greens to suit your taste preferences and nutritional needs. Feel free to swap spinach for kale or mix in other fruits like avocado, cucumber, or apple.

- If you prefer a thicker consistency, use less almond milk or add additional frozen fruit to the blender.

- Customise your toppings based on what you have available and what you enjoy. Incorporate a mix of textures and flavours for a well-rounded experience.

- Green smoothie bowls are not only tasty but also packed with vitamins, minerals, fibre, and antioxidants, making them a nutritious way to start your day or refuel after a workout.

- Get creative and have fun with your green smoothie bowl creations. Whether you're making them for breakfast, a post-workout snack, or a refreshing treat, they're sure to be a hit!

Avocado Toast with Tomato and Basil

Avocado toast with tomato and basil is a simple yet flavorful dish that's perfect for any meal of the day. Here's how to make it:

Ingredients:
- 1 ripe avocado

- 2 slices of whole grain bread (or bread of your choice)
- 1 medium tomato, thinly sliced
- Fresh basil leaves
- Salt and pepper to taste
- Optional toppings: red pepper flakes, balsamic glaze, hemp seeds, nutritional yeast, etc.

Instructions:

1. Toast the Bread:
   - Toast the slices of bread until they reach your desired level of crispiness.

2. Prepare the Avocado:
   - Cut the ripe avocado in half and remove the pit. Scoop out the flesh into a bowl and mash it with a fork until smooth. Season with salt and pepper to taste.

3. Assemble the Toast:
   - Spread a generous layer of mashed avocado onto each slice of toasted bread.

4. Add Tomato and Basil:
   - Arrange the thinly sliced tomato on top of the mashed avocado.

- Tear fresh basil leaves and scatter them over the tomato slices.

5. Season and Serve:
    - Sprinkle a pinch of salt and pepper over the assembled avocado toast.
    - Optionally, add any other toppings of your choice, such as red pepper flakes, balsamic glaze, hemp seeds, or nutritional yeast.

6. Enjoy:
    - Serve the avocado toast immediately while the bread is still warm and the toppings are fresh. Enjoy a satisfying breakfast, light lunch, or snack.

Tips:

- Choose ripe avocados that yield slightly to gentle pressure when squeezed. They should be creamy and easy to mash.

- Use high-quality, fresh ingredients for the best flavour. Look for ripe, juicy tomatoes and fragrant basil leaves.

- Experiment with different variations by adding extra toppings like sliced cucumber, red onion, microgreens, or a drizzle of olive oil.

- For added protein and nutrition, consider serving the avocado toast alongside a side salad or a bowl of soup.

- Avocado toast with tomato and basil is not only delicious but also packed with healthy fats, vitamins, and antioxidants, making it a nutritious addition to a vegan fatty liver diet.

Chia Seed Pudding with Mixed Berries

Chia seed pudding with mixed berries is a delightful and nutritious dessert or breakfast option. Here's how to make it:

Ingredients:
- 1/4 cup chia seeds
- 1 cup almond milk or any plant-based milk of your choice
- 1-2 tablespoons maple syrup or agave syrup (adjust to taste)
- 1/2 teaspoon vanilla extract (optional)
- Mixed berries (such as strawberries, blueberries, raspberries, blackberries)
- Optional toppings: sliced almonds, shredded coconut, mint leaves, etc.

Instructions:
1. Mix Chia Seeds and Liquid:

o   In a mixing bowl or jar, combine the chia seeds, almond milk, maple syrup, and vanilla extract (if using). Stir well to combine all the ingredients.

2. Let it Set:
    o   Once everything is well mixed, cover the bowl or jar and refrigerate for at least 2 hours, or preferably overnight. This allows the chia seeds to absorb the liquid and thicken into a pudding-like consistency.

3. Prepare the Berries:
    o   Wash the mixed berries and pat them dry with a paper towel. If using strawberries, hull and slice them.

4. Assemble the Pudding:
    o   Once the chia seed pudding has set, give it a good stir to break up any clumps and ensure a smooth texture.
    o   Spoon the pudding into serving bowls or jars.
    o   Top the pudding with the mixed berries, arranging them evenly over the surface.

5. Add Toppings:

o   Optionally, sprinkle sliced almonds,
       shredded coconut, or fresh mint
       leaves over the mixed berries for
       added flavour and texture.

6. Serve and Enjoy:
   o   Chia seed pudding with mixed
       berries is best served chilled. Enjoy
       it as a refreshing and nutritious
       dessert, breakfast, or snack option.

Tips:

- Feel free to customise the sweetness of the
  pudding by adjusting the amount of maple
  syrup or agave syrup to suit your taste
  preferences.

- Experiment with different types of
  plant-based milk for varied flavours and
  textures. Coconut milk, oat milk, or hemp
  milk are all great options.

- Get creative with the toppings! Try adding
  other fruits, nuts, seeds, or even a drizzle of
  nut butter for extra flavour and nutrition.

- Chia seed pudding with mixed berries is rich
  in fibre, omega-3 fatty acids, and
  antioxidants, making it a nourishing addition
  to a vegan fatty liver diet.

CHAPTER SIX

Satisfying Vegan Lunch Recipes

Quinoa Salad with Roasted Vegetables

Quinoa salad with roasted vegetables is a hearty
and nutritious option for a vegan lunch. Here's how
to make it:

Ingredients:
- 1 cup quinoa, rinsed
- 2 cups water or vegetable broth
- Assorted vegetables for roasting (such as
  bell peppers, zucchini, cherry tomatoes, red
  onion, carrots, etc.)
- 2 tablespoons olive oil
- Salt and pepper to taste
- 1/4 cup fresh parsley, chopped
- Optional add-ins: chickpeas, diced avocado,
  toasted nuts or seeds, dried cranberries,
  etc.

For the dressing:
- 3 tablespoons olive oil
- 2 tablespoons balsamic vinegar
- 1 tablespoon Dijon mustard

- **1 clove garlic, minced**
- **Salt and pepper to taste**

Instructions:

1. Preheat the oven and prepare the vegetables:

   - Preheat the oven to 400°F (200°C).
   - Chop the assorted vegetables into bite-sized pieces and place them on a baking sheet lined with parchment paper.
   - Drizzle the vegetables with olive oil and season with salt and pepper. Toss to coat evenly.

2. Roast the vegetables:

   - Roast the vegetables in the preheated oven for 20-25 minutes, or until they are tender and slightly caramelised, stirring halfway through cooking.

3. Cook the quinoa:

   - In a medium saucepan, combine the rinsed quinoa and water or vegetable broth.
   - Bring the mixture to a boil, then reduce the heat to low, cover, and simmer for 15-20 minutes, or until

the quinoa is cooked and the liquid
is absorbed.

- Remove from heat and let it sit,
  covered, for 5 minutes. Fluff the
  quinoa with a fork.

4. Make the dressing:
   - In a small bowl, whisk together the
     olive oil, balsamic vinegar, Dijon
     mustard, minced garlic, salt, and
     pepper until well combined.

5. Assemble the salad:
   - In a large mixing bowl, combine the
     cooked quinoa, roasted vegetables,
     and chopped parsley.
   - Pour the dressing over the salad and
     toss gently to coat everything evenly.

6. Add optional toppings:
   - If desired, add in additional toppings
     such as chickpeas, diced avocado,
     toasted nuts or seeds, or dried
     cranberries for extra flavour and
     texture.

7. Serve:
   - Serve the quinoa salad with roasted
     vegetables immediately, or
     refrigerate it for later. Enjoy it warm

or chilled as a satisfying and nutritious vegan lunch option.

Tips:

- Feel free to customise the roasted vegetable selection based on your preferences or what's in season.

- Double the batch and store leftovers in an airtight container in the refrigerator for easy meal prep throughout the week.

- This quinoa salad with roasted vegetables is not only delicious but also packed with fibre, protein, vitamins, and minerals, making it a nourishing addition to a vegan diet, including a vegan fatty liver diet.

Lentil Soup with Spinach and Turmeric

Lentil soup with spinach and turmeric is a comforting and nutritious dish that's perfect for warming up on a chilly day. Here's how to make it:

Ingredients:
- 1 cup dried green or brown lentils, rinsed and drained
- 1 tablespoon olive oil
- 1 onion, diced
- 3 cloves garlic, minced

- 1 teaspoon ground turmeric
- 1 teaspoon ground cumin
- 1/2 teaspoon ground coriander
- 1/4 teaspoon cayenne pepper (optional, for heat)
- 4 cups vegetable broth
- 2 cups water
- 2 carrots, diced
- 2 stalks celery, diced
- 1 bay leaf
- Salt and pepper to taste
- 3 cups fresh spinach, roughly chopped
- Juice of 1 lemon
- Fresh parsley or cilantro, chopped (for garnish)

Instructions:

1. Sauté the aromatics:
   - In a large pot or Dutch oven, heat the olive oil over medium heat. Add the diced onion and cook until softened, about 5 minutes.
   - Add the minced garlic, ground turmeric, ground cumin, ground coriander, and cayenne pepper (if using). Cook for an additional 1-2 minutes, until fragrant.

2. Add the lentils and liquids:
    - Stir in the rinsed lentils, vegetable broth, water, diced carrots, diced celery, and bay leaf. Bring the mixture to a boil, then reduce the heat to low and let it simmer, partially covered, for 20-25 minutes, or until the lentils and vegetables are tender.

3. Season and wilt the spinach:
    - Season the soup with salt and pepper to taste. Stir in the chopped spinach and lemon juice, and let it simmer for an additional 5 minutes, or until the spinach is wilted and the flavours are well combined.

4. Adjust seasoning and serve:
    - Taste the soup and adjust the seasoning if necessary, adding more salt, pepper, or lemon juice as desired.
    - Ladle the lentil soup into bowls and garnish with fresh parsley or cilantro before serving.

5. Enjoy:
    - Serve the lentil soup with spinach and turmeric hot, accompanied by

crusty bread or your favourite grain
for a satisfying and nourishing meal.

Tips:

- You can customise this soup by adding
  other vegetables such as diced tomatoes,
  sweet potatoes, or bell peppers.
- For a creamier texture, you can blend a
  portion of the soup with an immersion
  blender before adding the spinach.
- Turmeric not only adds vibrant colour to the
  soup but also provides anti-inflammatory
  properties and a subtle earthy flavour.
- Leftover soup can be stored in an airtight
  container in the refrigerator for up to 4 days
  or frozen for longer-term storage. Reheat
  gently on the stove or in the microwave
  before serving.

Chickpea and Vegetable Stir-Fry

Chickpea and vegetable stir-fry is a flavorful and
satisfying vegan lunch option that's quick and easy
to make. Here's how to prepare it:

Ingredients:
- 1 can (15 ounces) chickpeas, drained and
  rinsed
- 2 tablespoons olive oil
- 2 cloves garlic, minced
- 1 small onion, thinly sliced

- 1 bell pepper, thinly sliced (any colour)
- 1 medium carrot, julienned or thinly sliced
- 1 cup broccoli florets
- 1 cup snow peas, trimmed
- 1 cup mushrooms, sliced
- 2 tablespoons soy sauce or tamari
- 1 tablespoon rice vinegar
- 1 tablespoon maple syrup or agave nectar
- 1 teaspoon sesame oil
- 1 teaspoon grated fresh ginger
- Cooked rice or quinoa, for serving
- Sesame seeds and chopped green onions, for garnish (optional)

Instructions:

1. Prepare the Chickpeas:
   - If using canned chickpeas, drain and rinse them under cold water. Pat them dry with a paper towel and set aside.

2. Sauté the Aromatics:
   - Heat the olive oil in a large skillet or wok over medium heat. Add the minced garlic and thinly sliced onion. Sauté for 2-3 minutes, or until the onion is translucent and fragrant.

3. Add the Vegetables:
   - Add the bell pepper, carrot, broccoli florets, snow peas, and mushrooms to the skillet. Stir-fry for 5-7 minutes,

or until the vegetables are
tender-crisp.

4. Add the Chickpeas:
    o   Add the chickpeas to the skillet with
        the vegetables. Stir to combine and
        heat through for an additional 2-3
        minutes.

5. Prepare the Sauce:
    o   In a small bowl, whisk together the
        soy sauce or tamari, rice vinegar,
        maple syrup or agave nectar,
        sesame oil, and grated ginger until
        well combined.

6. Combine and Serve:
    o   Pour the sauce over the chickpea
        and vegetable mixture in the skillet.
        Stir well to coat everything evenly
        with the sauce.
    o   Continue to cook for another 2-3
        minutes, allowing the flavours to
        meld together.
    o   Remove the skillet from heat and
        serve the chickpea and vegetable
        stir-fry hot, over cooked rice or
        quinoa.
    o   Garnish with sesame seeds and
        chopped green onions, if desired.

Tips:

- Feel free to customise the vegetables based on what you have on hand or your personal preferences. Other great options include snap peas, bok choy, cabbage, or baby corn.

- For added protein and flavour, you can sprinkle the stir-fry with chopped roasted peanuts or cashews before serving.

- Adjust the seasoning and sweetness of the sauce to suit your taste preferences by adding more soy sauce, maple syrup, or rice vinegar as needed.

- This chickpea and vegetable stir-fry is a versatile dish that can be enjoyed as a standalone meal or paired with other side dishes such as steamed greens or a fresh salad.

CHAPTER SEVEN

Flavorful Vegan Dinner Recipes

Stuffed Bell Peppers with Brown Rice and Black Beans

Stuffed bell peppers are a versatile and satisfying dish that can be enjoyed by vegans and non-vegans alike. Packed with wholesome ingredients like brown rice, black beans, and a variety of flavorful spices, these stuffed peppers make for a hearty and nutritious dinner option. Whether you're looking for a tasty weeknight meal or a dish to impress guests at your next dinner party, these stuffed bell peppers are sure to please.

Ingredients:

- 4 large bell peppers (any colour)
- 1 cup cooked brown rice
- 1 cup cooked black beans
- 1 small onion, diced
- 2 cloves garlic, minced
- 1 cup diced tomatoes
- 1 teaspoon cumin
- 1 teaspoon chilli powder
- Salt and pepper to taste
- 1/4 cup chopped fresh cilantro
- 1/2 cup vegan shredded cheese (optional)

Instructions:

1. Preheat the oven to 375°F (190°C) and lightly grease a baking dish.

2. Cut the tops off the bell peppers and remove the seeds and membranes. Place the peppers upright in the prepared baking dish and set aside.

3. In a large skillet, heat a tablespoon of oil over medium heat. Add the diced onion and minced garlic, and sauté until softened and fragrant, about 5 minutes.

4. Stir in the cooked brown rice, black beans, diced tomatoes, cumin, chilli powder, salt, and pepper. Cook for an additional 5 minutes, allowing the flavours to meld together.

5. Remove the skillet from heat and stir in the chopped cilantro. Taste and adjust seasoning as needed.

6. Spoon the rice and bean mixture evenly into each bell pepper until they are filled to the top.

7. If using vegan shredded cheese, sprinkle it on top of each stuffed pepper.

8. Cover the baking dish with aluminium foil and bake in the preheated oven for 25-30 minutes, or until the peppers are tender.

9. Remove the foil and bake for an additional 5 minutes to melt the cheese (if using) and lightly brown the tops of the peppers.

10. Once done, remove from the oven and let cool for a few minutes before serving.

11. Garnish with additional chopped cilantro, if desired, and serve hot.

12. Enjoy these delicious stuffed bell peppers with brown rice and black beans as a satisfying vegan dinner option!

Vegan Chili with Sweet Potatoes and Kale

Warm, comforting, and packed with flavour, this vegan chilli featuring sweet potatoes and kale is the perfect dish to cosy up with on chilly evenings. Loaded with nutritious ingredients like beans, vegetables, and spices, this hearty chilli is not only delicious but also incredibly satisfying. Whether you're serving it for a weeknight dinner or entertaining friends and family, this vegan chilli is sure to be a crowd-pleaser.

Ingredients:

- 1 tablespoon olive oil
- 1 onion, diced
- 3 cloves garlic, minced
- 1 medium sweet potato, peeled and diced
- 1 red bell pepper, diced
- 1 green bell pepper, diced
- 1 can (15 ounces) diced tomatoes
- 1 can (15 ounces) black beans, drained and rinsed
- 1 can (15 ounces) kidney beans, drained and rinsed
- 4 cups vegetable broth
- 2 cups chopped kale
- 2 teaspoons chilli powder
- 1 teaspoon cumin
- 1/2 teaspoon paprika
- Salt and pepper to taste
- Fresh cilantro, for garnish (optional)
- Avocado slices, for garnish (optional)

Instructions:

1. In a large pot or Dutch oven, heat the olive oil over medium heat. Add the diced onion and minced garlic, and sauté until softened and fragrant, about 5 minutes.

2. Add the diced sweet potato and bell peppers to the pot, and cook for an additional 5 minutes, stirring occasionally.

3. Stir in the diced tomatoes (with their juices),
    black beans, kidney beans, vegetable broth,
    chilli powder, cumin, paprika, salt, and
    pepper. Bring the chilli to a simmer.

4. Reduce the heat to low, cover the pot, and
    let the chilli simmer for 20-25 minutes, or
    until the sweet potatoes are tender.

5. Once the sweet potatoes are cooked
    through, stir in the chopped kale and cook
    for an additional 5 minutes, until the kale is
    wilted and tender.

6. Taste and adjust the seasoning, adding
    more salt and pepper if needed.

7. Ladle the vegan chilli into bowls and garnish
    with fresh cilantro and avocado slices, if
    desired.

8. Serve hot and enjoy this comforting vegan
    chilli with sweet potatoes and kale as a
    hearty dinner option!

Spaghetti Squash Pad Thai

Looking for a healthier twist on traditional Pad
Thai? This Spaghetti Squash Pad Thai recipe is a
delicious and nutritious alternative that's sure to
satisfy your cravings. By swapping out traditional
rice noodles for spaghetti squash, this dish

becomes lighter, lower in carbs, and packed with vitamins and minerals. With its vibrant flavours and crunchy texture, this Spaghetti Squash Pad Thai is bound to become a new favourite in your dinner rotation.

Ingredients:

- 1 medium spaghetti squash
- 2 tablespoons olive oil
- 2 cloves garlic, minced
- 1 red bell pepper, thinly sliced
- 1 carrot, julienned
- 1 cup bean sprouts
- 2 green onions, chopped
- 1/4 cup chopped peanuts
- 1/4 cup chopped fresh cilantro
- Lime wedges, for serving

For the sauce:

- 1/4 cup soy sauce or tamari (for gluten-free option)
- 2 tablespoons rice vinegar
- 2 tablespoons maple syrup or coconut sugar
- 1 tablespoon lime juice
- 1 tablespoon sriracha or chilli garlic sauce
- 1 teaspoon grated ginger
- 2 cloves garlic, minced

Instructions:

1. Preheat the oven to 400°F (200°C). Cut the spaghetti squash in half lengthwise and scoop out the seeds with a spoon. Place the squash halves cut-side down on a baking sheet lined with parchment paper. Bake for 30-40 minutes, or until the squash is tender and easily pierced with a fork.

2. While the spaghetti squash is baking, prepare the sauce. In a small bowl, whisk together the soy sauce, rice vinegar, maple syrup, lime juice, sriracha, grated ginger, and minced garlic. Set aside.

3. Once the spaghetti squash is cooked, remove it from the oven and let it cool slightly. Use a fork to scrape the flesh of the squash into spaghetti-like strands. Transfer the squash strands to a large bowl and set aside.

4. In a large skillet or wok, heat the olive oil over medium heat. Add the minced garlic and cook for 1-2 minutes, until fragrant.

5. Add the sliced red bell pepper and julienned carrot to the skillet. Cook for 3-4 minutes, until the vegetables are slightly softened.

6. Add the spaghetti squash strands to the skillet, along with the bean sprouts and

chopped green onions. Pour the sauce over the mixture and toss everything together until well combined. Cook for an additional 2-3 minutes, until heated through.

7. Remove the skillet from heat and sprinkle the chopped peanuts and fresh cilantro over the top of the Spaghetti Squash Pad Thai.

8. Serve hot, with lime wedges on the side for squeezing over the dish.

9. Enjoy this healthy and flavorful Spaghetti Squash Pad Thai as a satisfying meal option!

CHAPTER EIGHT

Irresistible Vegan Snack and Dessert Recipes

Baked Sweet Potato Chips

Craving a crunchy and satisfying snack that's also healthy and vegan-friendly? Look no further than these Baked Sweet Potato Chips! Made with just a few simple ingredients, these crispy chips are perfect for satisfying your snack cravings without any guilt. With their natural sweetness and satisfying crunch, these Baked Sweet Potato Chips are sure to become a favourite in your snack rotation.

Ingredients:

- 2 medium sweet potatoes, washed and peeled
- 2 tablespoons olive oil
- 1 teaspoon paprika
- 1/2 teaspoon garlic powder
- 1/2 teaspoon sea salt
- Freshly ground black pepper, to taste
- Optional: additional seasonings such as cayenne pepper, cinnamon, or rosemary

Instructions:

1. Preheat the oven to 375°F (190°C). Line a
    baking sheet with parchment paper or a
    silicone baking mat and set aside.

2. Using a sharp knife or a mandoline slicer,
    thinly slice the sweet potatoes into rounds,
    about 1/8 inch thick. The thinner the slices,
    the crispier the chips will be.

3. In a large bowl, toss the sweet potato slices
    with olive oil, paprika, garlic powder, sea
    salt, and black pepper until evenly coated.
    Feel free to add any additional seasonings
    of your choice at this stage.

4. Arrange the seasoned sweet potato slices in
    a single layer on the prepared baking sheet,
    making sure they are not overlapping.

5. Bake in the preheated oven for 15-20
    minutes, then flip the chips over using a
    spatula. Bake for an additional 10-15
    minutes, or until the chips are crispy and
    lightly golden brown around the edges.

6. Keep a close eye on the chips during the
    last few minutes of baking to prevent them
    from burning.

7. Once the chips are done baking, remove
    them from the oven and let them cool on the

baking sheet for a few minutes to crisp up further.

8. Transfer the baked sweet potato chips to a serving bowl or plate and enjoy them immediately as a tasty vegan snack.

9. Store any leftover chips in an airtight container at room temperature for up to 3 days. Enjoy them on their own or serve them with your favourite dip or hummus for an extra delicious treat!

10. These Baked Sweet Potato Chips are not only delicious but also nutritious, making them the perfect guilt-free snack for any occasion.

Fruit Salsa with Cinnamon Tortilla Chips

Fruit salsa with cinnamon tortilla chips is a delightful and refreshing dish that perfectly balances sweet and savoury flavours. Packed with nutrients and bursting with vibrant colours, this recipe is not only delicious but also supports a healthy vegan diet, making it an ideal choice for those looking to improve their liver health while enjoying flavorful meals.

Ingredients:

- 2 cups mixed fruits (such as diced mangoes, strawberries, kiwis, and pineapple)
- 1 tablespoon fresh lime juice
- 1 tablespoon maple syrup or agave nectar
- 1 tablespoon finely chopped fresh mint leaves
- 4–6 whole wheat or gluten-free tortillas
- 1 tablespoon coconut oil, melted
- 1 tablespoon cinnamon
- Pinch of salt

Instructions:

1. Preheat the oven to 350°F (175°C) and line a baking sheet with parchment paper.

2. In a mixing bowl, combine the diced fruits, lime juice, maple syrup or agave nectar, and chopped mint leaves. Gently toss the mixture until the fruits are evenly coated. Set aside to allow the flavours to meld.

3. In a small bowl, mix together the melted coconut oil, cinnamon, and a pinch of salt. Brush both sides of each tortilla with the cinnamon-coconut oil mixture.

4. Stack the tortillas on top of each other and cut them into wedges using a sharp knife or pizza cutter.

5. Arrange the tortilla wedges in a single layer on the prepared baking sheet. Bake in the preheated oven for 8-10 minutes, or until the chips are golden brown and crispy.

6. Remove the cinnamon tortilla chips from the oven and allow them to cool for a few minutes.

7. Serve the fruit salsa in a bowl alongside the cinnamon tortilla chips for dipping. Enjoy this refreshing and nutritious snack as a delightful addition to your vegan fatty liver diet!

Tip: Feel free to customise the fruit salsa with your favourite seasonal fruits for variety and added freshness. Additionally, you can adjust the sweetness level by adding more or less maple syrup or agave nectar to suit your taste preferences.

Vegan Chocolate Avocado Mousse

Indulge your sweet tooth guilt-free with this decadent yet health-conscious Vegan Chocolate Avocado Mousse. Creamy, rich, and satisfying, this dessert is not only delicious but also packed with nutrients from the avocado base. Perfect for satisfying cravings while sticking to a vegan and liver-friendly diet.

Ingredients:

- 2 ripe avocados, peeled and pitted
- 1/4 cup cocoa powder
- 1/4 cup maple syrup or agave nectar
- 1 teaspoon vanilla extract
- Pinch of salt
- Optional toppings: fresh berries, shredded coconut, chopped nuts

Instructions:

1. In a food processor or blender, combine the ripe avocados, cocoa powder, maple syrup or agave nectar, vanilla extract, and a pinch of salt.

2. Blend the ingredients until smooth and creamy, scraping down the sides of the bowl or blender as needed to ensure everything is well combined.

3. Taste the mousse and adjust the sweetness or cocoa powder to your liking, if necessary.

4. Once the mousse reaches your desired consistency and taste, transfer it to serving bowls or glasses.

5. Cover the bowls or glasses with plastic wrap and refrigerate for at least 30 minutes to allow the mousse to chill and set.

6. Before serving, garnish the mousse with
    your choice of toppings, such as fresh
    berries, shredded coconut, or chopped nuts,
    for added flavour and texture.

7. Serve the Vegan Chocolate Avocado
    Mousse chilled and enjoy the creamy,
    chocolatey goodness guilt-free!

Tip:

For an extra special treat, try adding a hint of
cinnamon or espresso powder to enhance the
flavour profile of the mousse. Additionally, you can
experiment with different toppings to create your
own unique variations based on personal
preferences.

PLANT-BASED FOODS FOR OPTIMAL LIVER HEALTH: THE BEST VEGAN FOODS FOR LIVER HEALTH

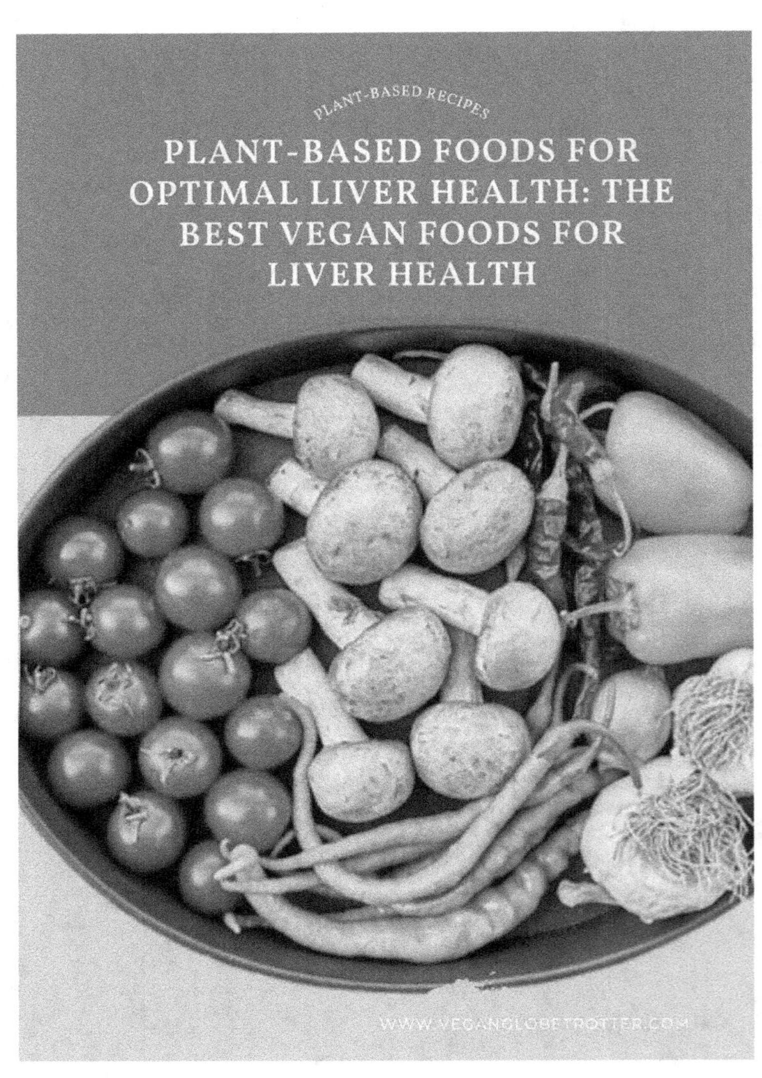

CHAPTER NINE

Lifestyle Tips for Supporting Liver Health

Importance of Exercise

Exercise plays a crucial role in supporting liver health and overall well-being. Here are some lifestyle tips highlighting the importance of exercise for maintaining a healthy liver:

1. **Promotes Weight Management:** Regular exercise helps to manage body weight by burning calories and reducing excess fat, which is essential for preventing obesity-related liver conditions such as fatty liver disease.

2. **Improves Insulin Sensitivity:** Physical activity enhances insulin sensitivity, which helps regulate blood sugar levels. This can lower the risk of developing insulin resistance and type 2 diabetes, both of which are risk factors for liver diseases.

3. **Enhances Blood Circulation:** Engaging in aerobic exercises like jogging, swimming, or cycling improves blood circulation throughout the body, including the liver.

Efficient blood flow supports liver function by delivering oxygen and nutrients while aiding in the removal of toxins.

4. **Reduces Inflammation:** Chronic inflammation is a common factor in many liver diseases. Regular exercise helps to reduce systemic inflammation by releasing anti-inflammatory cytokines, thereby protecting the liver from damage caused by inflammation.

5. **Lowers Risk of Non-Alcoholic Fatty Liver Disease (NAFLD):** NAFLD is strongly linked to sedentary behaviour and a lack of physical activity. Incorporating regular exercise into your routine can help prevent and manage NAFLD by reducing liver fat accumulation and improving liver function.

6. **Supports Detoxification:** Exercise stimulates the lymphatic system and promotes sweating, which aids in the elimination of toxins from the body. By supporting the body's natural detoxification processes, exercise assists the liver in removing harmful substances and maintaining optimal function.

7. **Boosts Immune Function:** Regular physical activity strengthens the immune system, making the body more resilient to

infections and illnesses. A healthy immune system is essential for protecting the liver from viral hepatitis and other infectious diseases that can cause liver damage.

8. **Improves Mental Health:** Exercise is known to boost mood, reduce stress, and alleviate symptoms of anxiety and depression. Mental well-being is closely linked to physical health, and maintaining a positive mindset can have a beneficial impact on liver function and overall health.

Incorporating regular exercise into your lifestyle, along with a balanced diet and other healthy habits, is key to supporting liver health and reducing the risk of liver diseases. Consult with a healthcare professional before starting any new exercise regimen, especially if you have existing health conditions or concerns.

Stress Management Techniques

Here are some stress management techniques as lifestyle tips for supporting liver health:

1. **Mindfulness Meditation:** Engage in mindfulness meditation to reduce stress levels and promote relaxation, which can positively impact liver function.

2. **Regular Exercise:** Incorporate regular physical activity into your routine to reduce stress hormones and improve overall well-being, which indirectly supports liver health.

3. **Healthy Diet:** Maintain a balanced diet rich in fruits, vegetables, whole grains, and lean proteins to provide essential nutrients for optimal liver function and combat stress-related inflammation.

4. **Adequate Sleep:** Prioritise quality sleep to allow your body and mind to rest and recharge, promoting better stress management and liver health.

5. **Stress-Reducing Activities:** Engage in activities you enjoy, such as hobbies, spending time with loved ones, or practising relaxation techniques like deep breathing exercises, to reduce stress levels and support liver health.

6. **Limit Alcohol Intake:** Excessive alcohol consumption can exacerbate stress on the liver. Limit alcohol intake or avoid it altogether to protect liver function and overall health.

7. **Time Management:** Organise your schedule effectively to avoid feeling overwhelmed, reducing stress levels and supporting liver health by preventing chronic stress.

8. **Social Support:** Seek support from friends, family, or support groups to share your feelings and experiences, which can help alleviate stress and promote liver health through emotional support.

9. **Limit Caffeine Intake:** While moderate caffeine consumption is generally safe, excessive caffeine intake can contribute to stress and anxiety. Limit caffeine intake to support overall stress management and liver health.

10. **Seek Professional Help:** If stress becomes overwhelming or difficult to manage on your own, consider seeking support from a therapist or counsellor who can provide coping strategies and support tailored to your needs.

By incorporating these stress management techniques into your lifestyle, you can not only reduce stress levels but also support liver health for overall well-being.

Sleep Hygiene and Its Impact on Liver Health

Sleep hygiene refers to a set of practices and habits that promote quality sleep. Here's how good sleep hygiene can positively impact liver health:

1. **Regulation of Circadian Rhythm:** Maintaining a consistent sleep schedule helps regulate your body's internal clock, known as the circadian rhythm. Disruptions in this rhythm, such as irregular sleep patterns or shift work, can negatively affect liver function by disrupting metabolic processes.

2. **Liver Detoxification:** During sleep, the liver undergoes a process of detoxification, eliminating toxins and waste products from the body. Adequate sleep duration and quality ensure that this detoxification process occurs efficiently, supporting optimal liver function.

3. **Reduced Risk of Non-Alcoholic Fatty Liver Disease (NAFLD):** Poor sleep habits, such as insufficient sleep duration or sleep disturbances, have been linked to an increased risk of developing NAFLD, a condition characterised by the accumulation of fat in the liver. By prioritising good sleep

hygiene, you can potentially lower your risk of NAFLD.

4. **Inflammation Reduction:** Quality sleep plays a crucial role in regulating inflammation levels in the body. Chronic sleep deprivation or poor sleep quality can lead to increased inflammation, which may contribute to liver inflammation and damage over time.

5. **Blood Sugar Regulation:** Sleep deprivation can disrupt glucose metabolism and insulin sensitivity, leading to higher blood sugar levels and an increased risk of developing conditions such as type 2 diabetes and fatty liver disease. Maintaining good sleep hygiene helps regulate blood sugar levels, thereby supporting liver health.

6. **Stress Reduction:** Adequate sleep is essential for managing stress levels. Chronic stress can negatively impact liver function by increasing inflammation and contributing to conditions such as non-alcoholic steatohepatitis (NASH). Prioritising sleep hygiene can help mitigate the effects of stress on the liver.

7. **Healthy Weight Maintenance:** Poor sleep habits have been associated with weight

gain and obesity, both of which are risk factors for NAFLD and other liver conditions. By promoting healthy weight maintenance, good sleep hygiene indirectly supports liver health.

To optimise sleep hygiene and promote liver health, consider implementing the following practices:

- Maintain a consistent sleep schedule by going to bed and waking up at the same time each day, even on weekends.

- Create a relaxing bedtime routine to signal to your body that it's time to wind down.

- Ensure your sleep environment is conducive to rest, with a comfortable mattress, supportive pillows, and a cool, dark, and quiet room.

- Limit exposure to screens (phones, computers, TVs) before bedtime, as the blue light emitted can interfere with melatonin production and disrupt sleep.

- Avoid consuming caffeine and large meals close to bedtime, as these can interfere with sleep quality.

CONCLUSION

In conclusion, the Vegan Fatty Liver Diet Cookbook serves as a comprehensive guide for individuals seeking to improve their liver health through plant-based nutrition. By embracing a vegan diet rich in fruits, vegetables, whole grains, legumes, nuts, and seeds, individuals can effectively manage and even reverse fatty liver disease while enjoying delicious and nutritious meals.

This cookbook goes beyond traditional dietary recommendations by offering flavorful recipes that are specifically tailored to support liver health. From vibrant salads and hearty soups to satisfying main dishes and indulgent desserts, each recipe is thoughtfully crafted to provide essential nutrients, antioxidants, and anti-inflammatory compounds that promote liver detoxification and function.

Furthermore, the Vegan Fatty Liver Diet Cookbook emphasises the importance of whole, unprocessed foods while minimising or eliminating added sugars, refined carbohydrates, and unhealthy fats. By focusing on nutrient-dense ingredients and mindful cooking techniques, individuals can optimise their nutritional intake and reduce the risk of exacerbating liver-related conditions.

Moreover, this cookbook acknowledges the diverse needs and preferences of its readers by offering a variety of recipes suitable for different dietary restrictions, including gluten-free, soy-free, and nut-free options. Whether you're new to veganism or a seasoned plant-based enthusiast, there's something for everyone to enjoy and benefit from in these pages.

Ultimately, the Vegan Fatty Liver Diet Cookbook empowers individuals to take control of their health and well-being through delicious, nourishing, and liver-friendly meals. By making simple yet impactful changes to their diet and lifestyle, readers can embark on a journey towards better liver health, increased vitality, and long-lasting wellness. With each recipe, they're not just nourishing their bodies—they're nurturing their liver and embracing a healthier, more vibrant way of living.